Nutrition

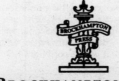

BROCKHAMPTON PRESS
LONDON

© 1996 Geddes & Grosset Ltd, David Dale House,
New Lanark ML11 9DJ.

This edition published 1996 by Brockhampton Press,
a member of Hodder Headline PLC Group.

ISBN 0 86019 292 0

Printed and bound in the UK

Introduction

Food is of fundamental importance to our lives as a source of energy to maintain life and as a means of enjoyment, relaxation and socializing. In the UK we are used to well-stocked shops and supermarkets that offer a wide variety of foods, and the majority of us are able to eat a diet that is adequate for our nutritional needs.

However, whilst the foods we include in our daily diet may meet our energy needs, they are not always the best choices we can make for our health and well-being. Much of the food that is now available and consumed in our society is highly refined and processed, and contains large amounts of sugar, salt, fat and artificial additives. The changes in our diet since the beginning of the century have been accompanied with the increased incidence of conditions such as heart disease, diverticulitis, bowel cancer, obesity and dental decay, which, after many years of research, have been significantly linked to dietary habits.

Obesity, which is fairly common in Western society, is caused in most cases by the consumption of too many foods that are high in fats and sugars. Research has shown that an obese person is more likely to develop heart disease, gall stones, arthritis and diabetes, whilst on an everyday level the extra weight makes basic activities harder for hime or her to perform and can have serious psychological effects.

Over the years there has been much advice about what a healthy diet should consist of, much of which has often been conflicting or confusing. Certainly, reducing our intake of fat and sugars to approximately 5 per cent of our daily intake and increasing the amount of wholegrains, fruit and vegetables we eat is basic, sound advice that is supported by the medical profession and nutritionists. However, balancing the diet can be more difficult; even if we know how much carbohydrate or protein we should eat, do we know why it is good for us and what it looks like? In the *Guide to Good Nutrition* we have provided information on all the major nutrients, vitamins and minerals—what they do, the amount we need, the foods from which they can be derived. We have also compiled a nutritional chart of basic foods, which specifically calculates the quantities of carbohydrates, proteins, fat, fibre and the number of calories in fruit, vegetables, meat, fish and seafood, cereals, nuts and seeds and beverages.

We have also included a section on nutrition and weight loss, which explains how weight is gained and lost and provides basic advice for permanently losing weight whilst maintaining adequate nutrition.

Healthy eating habits are not restrictive or boring. Even small adjustments to the the diet can be beneficial to our health without compromising our enjoyment of food. With the help of this book you will be able to establish a better understanding of the way in which food fuels the body and identify ways in which you can enjoy your favourite foods in the healthiest way.

Nutrients

There are six basic groups of nutrients: carbohydrate, protein and fat, which all provide energy, and vitamins, minerals and water, which do not provide the body with energy but are vital in assisting in the maintenance of the basic processes of the body; dietary fibre, included in this section, is not technically a nutrient but has been covered here because it is so important in establishing a healthy diet.

Carbohydrates

Carbohydrates are necessary for providing the body with energy and are vital for the maintenance of many of its metabolic functions and the complete burning of fat. Carbohydrates can be consumed in two forms—simple and complex. Most carbohydrates consumed should be in the complex form, which is found in grains, beans and starchy vegetables such as potatoes and root vegetables. These are not as easily converted into storage fat as other foods and tend to contain fibre.

Simple carbohydrates can be found in sugar form in highly processed, refined foods, and in this form tend to have a low nutritional value. However, fruit which contain the simple carbohydrate fructose is a valuable source of vitamins, minerals and fibre.

It is recommended that carbohydrates constitute 55 to 60 per cent of the daily dietary intake.

Protein

Protein is essential for the development and maintenance of body tissue and the growth and repair cells. Proteins are made up of amino acids, some of which cannot be synthesized or manufactured by the human body and, therefore, must be derived from diet. Foods that supply *all* amino acids are meat, fish, eggs, cheese and milk. Protein foods derived from plant origin, such as cereals, pulses, nuts and seeds, do not contain all the essential amino acids but remain a relatively valuable source of protein if two protein types are eaten together; for example, pulses and cereals. The average recommended daily amounts of protein are 54g for an adult woman and 63g for an adult man. The average British diet tends to have a higher protein content than is really necessary, and it is recommended that essential amino acids are taken from low-fat sources such as the white meat of chicken and turkey, fish, low-fat dairy products, lean cuts of meats and vegetable sources.

Fats

Fats are necessary in a diet; along with carbohydrates they are the main dietary source for maintaining base metabolism. Fats are also necessary for the absorption of the fat-soluble vitamins A, D, E and K, for the formation of the outer protective covering of the nerves and for the maintenance of cell membranes. Some fatty acids cannot be synthesized by the body and, therefore, must be included in the diet. However, it is recommended that these should be taken mainly in the form of monounsaturated and polyunsaturated fats, which are derived from plant sources. Saturated fat, found in meat and many dairy products such as butter, cream and cheese, is associated with the development of cholesterol, high levels of which can cause a hardening of the arteries leading to heart disease.

Water

Water is essential for health. It is vital for the transportation of nutrients and other material around the body, for maintaining the chemical balance of the body and for the excretion of waste products. The minimum recommended daily intake of water is approximately 1500ml, some of which should be taken in the form of tap or bottled water. It can also be taken in the form of hot drinks such as tea and coffee, fizzy drinks, fruit juice and from solid foods such as fruit and vegetables, which are composed mainly of water.

Fibre

Whilst not an essential nutrient, fibre is important in maintaining a healthy diet. Dietary fibre is found in the cell walls of plant foods and cannot be digested by humans. Western diets, which have a high content of refined, processed foods, tend to be lacking in dietary fibre; conditions of the large intestine such as diverticulitis, constipation and bowel cancer are more common in societies where the intake of fibre tends to be low.

Fibre is advantageous for a healthy diet since many of the foods that are high in fibre are also low in fat. Fibre is also very filling and absorbs water, assisting the easy passage of faeces through the bowel.

The recommended daily amount of dietary fibre is at least 30g and can be derived from wholegrain cereal foods, such as wholemeal bread and low-sugar breakfast cereals, fruit, vegetables and pulses.

Vitamins

Vitamins are essential for health and can be easily supplied through a varied and balanced diet as they are needed only in small amounts.

Vitamins can be divided into two main groups; fat-soluble vitamins (A, D, E and K) and water-soluble vitamins (the B group of vitamins and vitamin C). Unlike fat-soluble vitamins, water-soluble vitamins are not stored by the body and can be lost from food through the processes of storing, preparation and cooking. It is therefore necessary to ensure that adequate amounts of the water-soluble vitamins are included in the daily diet.

Vitamin A

Vitamin A is important for normal growth in children, for maintaining the condition of skin and mucous membranes and for aiding vision in poor light. It occurs in animal foods as retinol, and sources include liver, butter, margarine, cheese, egg yolk and milk. In plant foods it occurs as carotene and can be converted to retinol in the body. Good sources of carotene include carrots, tomatoes, spinach, watercress and dried apricots. The recommended daily allowance of vitamin A is 750 micrograms for adults and 300–725 micrograms a day for children aged up to 14 years. For pregnant and lactating women the recommended daily intake is 1200 micrograms.

Vitamin D (cholecalciferol)

Vitamin D is essential for the absorption and metabolism of calcium in the diet. A deficiency of cholecalciferol would lead to rickets in children and tenderness and weakness in the bones of adults, known as osteomalacia. The main food sources of vitamin D are halibut and cod liver oil, oily fish, egg yolk, butter, cheese, margarine and milk. Vitamin D can also be obtained from the effect sunlight has on a substance beneath the skin called dehydrocholesterol.

The recommended daily intake of vitamin D is 2.5 micrograms for an adult, although generally a sufficient supply can be provided by sunlight. However, young children and pregnant women should also receive a dietary intake since the requirements for the formation of bones and teeth will be greater.

Vitamin E (tocopherol)

There is no specific function of vitamin E that has, as yet, been identified, and a deficiency is unknown because it available from so many food sources. Foods rich in vitamin E include cereals, green vegetable leaves, vegetable oils and milk.

Vitamin K

Vitamin K is an essential factor in maintaining the clotting mechanism of the blood and is available from all foods, green leafy vegetables and peas being particularly rich sources. There is no recommendation for the daily intake of vitamin K as a deficiency in the diet is very rare.

Vitamin B$_1$ (thiamin)

Vitamin B$_1$ is required to maintain the steady, continuous release of energy from carbohydrates, and is available from bread, flour, pork, potatoes, brewer's yeast and many fortified wheatgerm breakfast cereals. The daily requirement of vitamin B$_1$ is related to the amount of carbohydrate in a diet, although a basic requirement for adults can be given as 1.2 mg. Severe deficiency is rare

in developed countries, although symptoms such as
inflammation of the nerves, depression and irritability
can occur if a diet rich in carbohydrate is deficient in
vitamin B_1

Vitamin B_2 (riboflavin)

A deficiency of vitamin B_2 is rare as it is widely available
in yeast, dairy products, milk, eggs and liver. However, a
lack of vitamin B_2 will affect the mucosal lining of the
mouth, leading to cracks in the skin around the mouth
and the tongue. The recommended daily intake is
approximately 1.7 mg in an adult.

Vitamin B_3 (nicotinic acid)

Nicotinic acid is involved in the process of metabolizing
the energy derived from food and is widely available
from many sources, including meat, yeast, flour, fortified
breakfast cereals, vegetables, milk and eggs. A deficiency
in nicotinic acid is rare, but symptoms can include
diarrhoea and a change in the condition of the skin. A
basic intake of 18 mg a day is recommended for adults.

Vitamin B_6 (pyridoxine)

Pyridoxine is associated with the metabolism of proteins
and is present in most foods.

Folic acid and vitamin B_{12}

Folic acid is essential for assisting in the formation of
red blood cells and is available from yeast, dark green
vegetables and liver, although it can be destroyed during
preparation and cooking. A deficiency can cause a form
of anaemia. Vitamin B_{12} is also essential for the
development of red blood cells and can be supplied by
the streptomycin cultures from liver and dark green
vegetables. It is also synthesized by bacteria in the
intestines and so deficiency is rare.

Vitamin C (ascorbic acid)

Ascorbic acid is necessary for the effective formation
and maintenance of connective tissue and for the healthy
development of bones and teeth. Ascorbic acid is found
in pure fruit juices, citrus fruits, blackcurrants, new
potatoes, tomatoes and green leaf vegetables. However,
it can be lost if fresh fruit and vegetables are stored over
a long time and through some preparation and cooking
techniques. The recommended daily intake is 20–30mg
for children, 30mg for adults and 60mg for pregnant and
breastfeeding women.

Minerals

Minerals are essential as constituents of bone tissue and
body fluid, in the transmission of nerve impulses and
the control of the release and metabolism of energy. The
major minerals are calcium and phosphorus, iron,
magnesium, sodium and potassium, and iodine.

Calcium and phosphorus

Calcium and phosphorus are both found in bone tissue
as calcium phosphate, the substance that maintains the
strength of bones and teeth. Calcium also plays an
important role in blood clotting and in maintaining the
function of muscles and nerves. It can be derived from
milk, cheese and bread and in fortified flour. Strict
vegans may be at risk from deficiency, which in later life
can lead to a weakening and thinning of the bones,
known as osteoporosis. The recommended daily intake
is 500mg, although growing children and breastfeeding
women may require more.

Phosphorus is present in most foods and is often
added to processed foods.

Iron

Iron is an essential element of haemoglobin, which enables red blood cells to transport oxygen around the body; anaemia is typically associated with a deficiency of iron. The richest sources of iron are red meat and liver, which are easily absorbed. Egg yolk, dark green leaf vegetables, dried apricots and fortified breakfast cereals and flours are also good sources. The recommended daily intake is 10–12mg a day, although pregnant and menstruating women require more iron than men.

Magnesium

Magnesium is an essential element in the metabolism of carbohydrates and for the transmission of nerve signals to muscles. Primary dietary sources of magnesium include milk, nuts, wholegrain cereals, broad beans and peas. The recommended daily intake is 300–500mg and deficiency is rare.

Sodium and potassium

Sodium and potassium are present in all body fluids and are necessary in maintaining the fluid balance of the body. When taken in the diet both minerals are absorbed, and any excess is excreted in urine. However, in cases of damage or disease of the kidney the intake of both will need to be restricted; babies should never have sodium or potassium added to their food.

Sodium is available as salt, added when cooking, used at the table or found in many processed foods. The daily requirement is 1 gram a day. The average intake in the UK is five to ten times higher, and it is recommended that to avoid developing high blood pressure the amount we take is reduced. Potassium is available in vegetables, fruit, meat and milk, and deficiency is unlikely.

Iodine

Iodine is important for efficiently maintaining metabolism as it is a constituent of the hormone thyroxine, which is released from the thyroid gland, situated in the neck. A deficiency of iodine would cause goitre, a swelling of the thyroid gland. Rich sources of iodine include iodized table salt and seafood. Whilst iodine can be found in fruit and vegetables the amount may vary as some soils have a low iodine content. However, iodine is needed in such small amounts that deficiency rarely occurs.

Nutrition and weight reduction

Through medical research it has been suggested that a tendency to be overweight can be genetically inherited. Certainly, the distribution of fat in our bodies can be passed on; rather like our facial features, our body shape can resemble that of our parents and relatives. However, irrespective of the fat cells we may be born with, diet generally remains the most important factor in determining our adult weight.

As an adult, excess weight is gained when we exceed our bodily energy requirements through our daily intake of food and fluid. It is estimated that the average daily energy requirement for an adult woman is approximately equal to 2000 calories. If the daily dietary intake consistently exceeds this then the excess energy not utilized by the body will be stored as fat cells, and weight will be gained.

Conversely, weight is lost if the daily intake of calories is lower than the energy requirements of the body. To meet the energy deficit the body will draw on triglycerides, which are energy efficient chemicals that are stored in the fat cells of the body; the fat cells will then shrink, and weight loss will result.

The body's energy requirement is dependent on various factors, including height, weight and sex. On average we need between 1150 and 2015 calories for the body to be able to maintain its basic functions, such as circulation, respiration, the regulation of body temperature and cell regeneration. The rate at which these vital processes use energy is called the basal metabolic rate and requires between 0.8 and 1.4 calories per minute. Basic physical activity, even sitting and sleeping, requires energy and so the daily physical activity in which an individual is involved will also be a factor determining the daily calorific requirement.

To lose 0.5 kg in weight necessitates using 3500 more calories than are consumed in food. So for the average woman with a basic calorie requirement of 2000 calories per day, reducing the calorie intake to 1500 calories per day would result in an average weight loss of 0.5kg a week. Depending, again, on height, weight, sex and physical activity, women should try to maintain a calorific intake of 1000–1500 calories per day and men 1500–2000 calories to achieve a gradual weight loss. Those with more weight to lose should set their intake at the higher end of these ranges since their weight loss programme will take longer.

Rapid weight loss associated with the highly restrictive calorific intake of crash dieting is not advisable. Whilst it may be more encouraging for the individual to lose weight quickly, it is difficult to maintain over a long period of time and is likely to result in an eventual regain of the lost weight.

If the body receives fewer than 1000 calories a day over a sustained period it will respond by lowering the basal metabolic rate, requiring less and less energy to perform the basic functions. Once the calorie intake is increased again the body will respond by storing excess energy as fat cells.

On a highly restrictive diet it is also very difficult to ensure that an adequate state of nutrition is maintained. When trying to lose weight it is important that sufficient carbohydrate, protein, fat, fibre, vitamins and minerals are still supplied in the diet. For example, a high-protein diet that restricts the intake of carbohydrates will initially result in a rapid weight loss, most of which will be water as opposed to body fat. As the diet progresses there is a large build-up of waste products (because carbohydrates are necessary for the complete burning of body fat), which will again be excreted in water. When carbohydrates are reintroduced to the diet, the body readjusts and much of the lost weight will be gained.

Succesful and permanent weight loss lies in changing eating habits and adopting a more healthy approach to diet. The most significant change that can be made is cutting down on the amount of fat consumed. By weight, fats contain twice as many calories as carbohydrates and proteins, and only a small amount is actually needed by the body for nutritional purposes. Saturated fats, derived from animal sources, have been significantly linked to heart disease, and it is recommended by dietitians and the medical profession that fats should be derived mainly from vegetable sources.

Reducing consumption of red meat, using polyunsaturated margarines instead of butter and animal fat margarines, cooking with vegetable oils and using skimmed or semi-skimmed milk instead of whole milk are all changes that can be easily and permanently made.

Combining diet with exercise is the most effective method for permanent weight loss. Increasing physical activity will burn up more calories, allowing a more rapid weight loss and a less restrictive calorific intake. Exercise also increases the percentage of body fat lost in relation to lean muscle tissue. A weight loss programme that depends solely on calorie reduction can result in the loss of lean tissue as well as fat. An exercise programme will help to ensure that significantly more body fat than lean tissue is lost.

Average recommended daily energy intake

	Energy Kilocalories
Children, age 1–2	1100–1400
Children, age 3–4	1500–1560
Children, age 5–6	1680–1740
Children, age 7–8	1900–1980
Teenagers	2150–2800
Women, age 18–54 (sedentary)	2150
Women, age 18–54 (very active)	2300–2500
Pregnant and lactating women	2400–2750
Men, age 18–54 (sedentary)	2500–2700
Men, age 18–54 (very active)	2800–3500

Desirable Weights for Adults

Height (m)	Men (kg)	Women (kg)
1.42		41–45
1.45		42–53
1.48		42–54
1.50		43–55
1.52		44–57
1.54		44–58
1.56		45–58
1.58	51–64	46–59
1.60	52–65	49–61
1.62	53–66	49–62
1.64	54–67	50–64
1.66	54–69	51–65
1.68	56–71	52–66
1.70	58–73	53–67
1.72	59–74	55–69
1.74	60–75	56–70
1.76	62–77	58–72
1.78	64–79	59–74
1.80	65–80	
1.82	66–82	
1.84	67–84	
1.86	69–86	
1.88	71–88	
1.90	73–90	
1.92	75–93	

Nutritional guide to basic foods

Fruit

Specific	Amount	Kcals	Carb	Prot	Fat	Fibre
Apples						
cooking, raw, peeled	100g	35	8.9	0.3	0.1	2.2
eating, raw, with core	100g	42	10.5	0.4	0.1	1.8
eating, raw, with core	1 small [75g]	32	7.9	0.3	0.1	1.6
eating, raw, with core	1 medium [112g]	47	11.8	0.4	0.1	2.0
eating, raw, with core	1 large [170g]	71	17.9	0.7	0.2	3.0
eating, raw, peeled	100g	45	11.2	0.4	0.1	1.8
Apricots						
raw, without stone	100g	31	8.5	0.3	0.1	1.9
raw, without stone	1 [65g]	20	5.5	0.2	0.1	1.2
semi-dried, ready-to-eat	100g	158	36.5	4.0	0.6	18.1
Avocado						
raw, without skin or stone	100g	190	1.9	1.9	19.5	3.4
raw, without skin or stone	1 small [100g]	190	1.9	1.9	19.5	3.4
raw, without skin or stone	1 medium [145g]	275	2.8	2.8	28.3	4.9
raw, without skin or stone	1 large [195g]	371	3.7	3.7	38.0	6.6
Banana						
with skin	100g	95	23.2	1.2	0.3	3.0
with skin	1 small [130g]	123	30.2	1.6	0.4	3.9
with skin	1 medium [150g]	143	34.8	1.8	0.5	4.5
with skin	1 large [180g]	171	41.8	2.2	0.5	5.4

Specific	Amount	Kcals	Carb	Prot	Fat	Fibre
Blackberries						
raw	100g	25	5.1	0.9	0.2	6.6
Blackcurrants						
raw	100g	28	6.6	0.9	trace	7.8
Cherries						
raw, without stone	100g	48	11.5	0.9	0.1	1.5
Clementines						
raw, without skin	100g	37	8.7	0.9	0.1	1.7
raw, without skin	1 small [40g]	15	3.5	0.4	trace	0.7
raw, without skin	1 medium [60g]	22	5.2	0.5	0.1	1.0
raw, without skin	1 large [80g]	30	7.0	0.7	0.1	1.4
Currants	100g	267	67.8	2.3	0.4	5.9
Damsons						
raw, without stones	100g	34	8.6	0.5	trace	3.3
raw, without stones	1 [15g]	5	1.3	trace	trace	0.5
Dates						
dried, with stones	100g	227	57.1	2.8	0.2	6.5
dried, with stone	1 [20g]	45	11.4	0.6	trace	1.3
raw, with stones	100g	107	26.9	1.3	0.1	3.1
raw, with stone	1 [30g]	32	8.1	0.4	trace	0.9
Figs						
dried	100g	227	52.9	3.6	1.6	12.4
dried	1 [20g]	45	10.6	0.7	0.3	2.5
semi-dried, ready-to-eat	100g	209	48.6	3.3	1.5	11.4

Specific	Amount	Kcals	Carb	Prot	Fat	Fibre
semi-dried, ready-to-eat	1 [35g]	73	17.0	1.2	0.5	4.0
Gooseberries						
cooking, raw	100g	19	3.0	1.1	0.4	2.9
Grapefruit						
raw, with skin	100g	20	4.6	0.5	0.1	1.1
raw, with skin	1 small [250g]	50	11.5	1.3	0.3	2.8
raw, with skin	1 medium [340g]	68	15.6	1.7	0.3	3.7
raw, with skin	1 large [425g]	85	19.6	2.1	0.4	4.7
Grapes						
raw, black and white	100g	60	15.4	0.4	0.1	0.8
raw, black and white	1 [5g]	3	0.8	trace	trace	trace
Guava						
raw	100g	26	5.0	0.8	0.5	4.7
Kiwi fruit						
raw, without skin	100g	49	10.6	1.1	0.5	1.9
raw, without skin	1 [60g]	29	6.3	0.7	0.3	1.1
Lemons						
raw, with peel	100g	19	3.2	1.0	0.3	4.7
raw, with peel	1 medium [125g]	24	4.0	1.3	0.3	5.9
Lychees						
raw, without stone	100g	58	14.3	0.9	0.1	1.5
raw, without stone	1 [15g]	9	2.1	0.1	trace	0.2
Mandarin oranges						
raw, without peel	100g	35	8.7	0.9	0.1	1.2

Specific	Amount	Kcals	Carb	Prot	Fat	Fibre
raw with peel	1 medium [75g]	26	6.5	0.7	0.1	0.9
Mangoes						
raw, without stone or skin	100g	57	14.1	0.7	0.2	2.9
raw, without stone or skin	1 slice [40g]	23	5.6	0.3	trace	1.2
Melon						
Canteloupe, without skin or seeds	100g	19	4.2	0.6	0.1	0.9
Canteloupe, without skin or seeds	1 slice [150g]	29	6.3	0.9	0.2	1.3
Galia, without skin or seeds	100g	24	5.6	0.5	0.1	0.9
Galia, without skin or seeds	1 slice [150g]	36	8.4	0.8	0.2	1.3
Honeydew, without skin or seeds	100g	28	6.6	0.6	0.1	0.8
Honeydew, without skin or seeds	1 slice [180g]	50	11.8	1.1	0.2	1.4
Watermelon, without skin or seeds	100g	31	7.1	0.5	0.3	0.3
Watermelon, without skin or seeds	1 slice [200g]	62	14.2	1.0	0.6	0.6
Nectarines						
raw, without stones	100g	40	9.0	1.4	0.1	2.2
raw, without stone	1 small [125g]	50	11.3	1.8	0.1	2.8
raw, without stone	1 medium [140g]	56	12.6	2.0	0.1	3.1
raw, without stone	1 large [175g]	70	15.8	3.5	0.2	3.9
Olives						
in brine, without stones	100g	103	trace	0.9	11.0	4.0
Oranges						
raw, without skin	100g	37	8.5	1.1	0.1	1.8
raw, without skin	1 small [120g]	46	10.6	1.4	0.1	4.4
raw, without skin	1 medium [160g]	59	13.6	2.2	0.2	2.9

Specific	Amount	Kcals	Carb	Prot	Fat	Fibre
raw, without skin	1 large [210g]	78	17.9	2.3	2.2	3.8
Passion fruit						
raw, without skin	100g	36	5.8	2.6	0.4	3.3
raw, without skin	1 [15g]	5	0.9	0.4	trace	0.5
Peaches						
raw, without stone	100g	33	7.6	1.0	0.1	2.3
raw, without stone	1 small [70g]	23	5.3	0.7	trace	1.6
raw, without stone	1 medium [110g]	36	8.4	1.1	0.1	2.5
raw, without stone	1 large [150g]	50	11.4	1.5	0.2	3.4
Pears						
raw, without core	100g	40	10.0	0.3	0.1	2.2
raw, without core	1 medium [200g]	80	20.0	0.6	0.2	4.4
raw, peeled	100g	41	10.4	0.3	0.1	2.7
Pineapple						
raw, without skin	100g	41	10.1	0.4	0.2	1.3
raw, without skin	1 slice [80g]	33	8.1	0.3	0.2	1.0
Plums						
raw, without stone	100g	34	8.3	0.5	0.1	2.3
raw, without stone	1 small [30g]	10	2.5	0.2	trace	0.7
raw, without stone	1 medium [55g]	19	4.6	0.3	0.1	1.3
raw, without stone	1 large [85g]	29	7.1	0.4	0.1	2.0
Prunes						
semi-dried, ready-to-eat	100g	141	34.0	2.5	0.4	12.8
semi-dried, ready-to-eat	1 [15g]	21	5.1	0.4	trace	1.9

Specific	Amount	Kcals	Carb	Prot	Fat	Fibre
Raisins	100g	272	69.3	2.1	0.4	6.9
	1 tbsp [30g]	82	20.8	0.6	trace	1.8
Raspberries						
raw	100g	25	4.6	1.4	0.3	6.7
Rhubarb						
raw	100g	7	0.8	0.9	0.1	2.3
Satsumas						
raw, without peel	100g	36	8.5	0.9	0.1	1.7
raw, without peel	1 small [50g]	18	4.3	0.5	0.1	0.9
raw, without peel	1 medium [70g]	25	6.0	0.6	0.1	1.2
raw, without peel	1 large [90g]	32	7.7	0.8	0.1	1.5
Strawberries						
raw	100g	27	6.0	0.8	0.1	2.0
raw	1 [12g]	3	6.1	0.1	trace	0.2
Sultanas	100g	275	69.4	2.7	0.4	6.3
	1 tbsp [30g]	83	20.8	0.8	trace	1.9
Tangerines						
raw	100g	35	8.0	0.9	0.1	1.7
raw	1 small [50g]	18	4.0	0.5	0.1	0.9
raw	1 medium [70g]	25	5.6	0.6	0.1	1.2
raw	1 large [90g]	32	7.2	0.6	0.1	1.5

Vegetables

Specific	Amount	Kcals	Carb	Prot	Fat	Fibre
Asparagus						
boiled	100g	26	1.4	3.4	0.8	1.4
boiled	5 spears [125g]	33	1.7	4.3	1.0	1.8
raw	100g	25	2.0	2.9	0.6	1.7
Aubergine						
fried in corn oil	100g	302	2.8	1.2	31.9	2.9
raw	100g	15	2.2	0.9	0.4	2.3
Bamboo Shoots						
canned, drained	100g	39	9.7	0.7	0	1.0
canned, drained	225g can	88	21.8	1.6	0	2.3
Beans						
Aduki, dried, boiled	100g	123	22.5	9.3	0.2	5.5
Aduki, dried, boiled	1 tbsp [30g]	37	6.8	2.8	trace	1.7
Baked, canned in tomato sauce	100g	84	15.3	5.2	0.6	6.9
Baked, canned in tomato sauce	1 tbsp [45g]	38	6.9	2.3	0.3	3.1
Blackeye, dried, boiled	100g	116	19.9	8.8	0.7	3.5
Blackeye, dried, boiled	1 tbsp [45g]	52	10.7	4	trace	1.6
Broad, frozen, boiled	100g	81	11.7	7.9	0.6	6.5
Butter, dried, boiled	100g	95	17	6.5	0.4	7.5
French, frozen, boiled	100g	25	4.7	1.7	0.1	4.1
French, raw	100g	24	3.2	1.9	0.5	2.2

Specific	Amount	Kcals	Carb	Prot	Fat	Fibre
Mung, dried, boiled	100g	91	15.3	7.6	0.4	4.8
Mung, dried, boiled	1 tbsp [30g]	27	4.6	2.3	0.1	1.4
Red kidney, dried, boiled	100g	103	17.4	8.4	0.5	9.0
Red kidney, dried, boiled	1 tbsp [30g]	31	5.2	2.5	0.2	2.7
Runner, boiled	100g	186	2.3	1.2	0.5	3.1
Runner, raw	100g	22	3.2	1.6	0.4	2.6
Soya, dried, boiled	100g	141	5.1	14.0	7.3	6.1
Soya, dried, boiled	1 tbsp [30g]	42	1.5	4.2	2.2	1.8
Beansprouts						
Mung, raw	100g	31	4.0	2.9	0.5	5.6
Beetroot						
boiled	100g	46	9.5	2.3	0.1	2.3
boiled	1 slice [10g]	5	1.0	0.2	trace	0.2
pickled, drained	100g	28	5.6	1.2	0.2	2.5
pickled, drained	1 slice [10g]	3	0.6	0.1	trace	0.3
raw	100g	36	7.6	1.7	0.1	2.8
Black gram	100g	89	13.6	7.8	0.4	5.8
Broccoli						
boiled	100g	24	1.1	3.1	0.8	2.3
raw	100g	33	1.8	4.4	0.9	2.6
Brussels sprouts						
boiled	100g	35	3.5	2.9	1.3	2.6
frozen, boiled	100g	35	2.5	3.5	1.3	4.0
raw	100g	42	4.1	5.3	1.4	3.8

Specific	Amount	Kcals	Carb	Prot	Fat	Fibre
Cabbage						
boiled	100g	18	2.5	0.8	0.6	2.5
raw	100g	26	4.1	1.7	0.4	2.9
white, raw	100g	27	5.0	1.4	0.2	2.4
Carrots						
old, boiled	100g	24	4.9	0.6	0.4	2.8
old, raw	100g	35	2.5	0.3	0.2	2.6
young, boiled	100g	22	4.4	0.6	0.4	2.7
young, raw	100g	30	6.0	0.7	0.5	2.6
Cauliflower						
boiled	100g	28	2.1	2.9	0.9	1.6
raw	100g	34	3.0	3.6	0.9	1.9
raw	1 floret [10g]	3	0.3	0.4	trace	0.2
Celery						
boiled	100g	8	0.8	0.5	0.3	2.0
raw	100g	7	0.9	0.5	0.2	1.6
raw	1 stick [30g]	2	0.3	0.2	0.1	0.5
Chick peas						
dried, boiled	100g	121	18.2	8.4	2.1	4.8
Chicory						
raw	100g	11	2.8	0.5	0.6	0.9
Courgette						
boiled	100g	19	2.0	2.0	0.4	1.2
raw	100g	18	1.8	1.8	0.4	0.9

Specific	Amount	Kcals	Carb	Prot	Fat	Fibre
Cucumber						
raw	100g	10	1.5	0.7	0.1	0.7
raw	1 inch piece [60g]	6	0.9	0.4	0.1	0.4
Curly Kale						
boiled	100g	24	1.0	2.4	1.1	2.6
raw	100g	33	1.4	3.4	1.6	3.3
Fennel						
boiled	100g	11	1.5	0.9	0.2	2.3
raw	100g	12	1.8	0.9	0.2	2.4
Garlic						
raw	100g	98	16.3	7.9	0.6	4.1
Gherkins						
pickled, drained	100g	14	2.6	0.9	0.1	1.2
Gourd						
raw	100g	11	0.8	1.6	0.2	3.6
Leeks						
boiled	100g	21	2.6	1.2	0.7	2.4
boiled	1, medium [160g]	34	4.2	1.9	1.1	3.8
raw	100g	22	2.9	1.6	0.5	2.8
Lentils						
green and brown, whole, dried and boiled	100g	105	16.9	8.8	0.7	3.8
green and brown, whole boiled	1 tbsp [30g]	32	5.1	2.6	0.2	1.1

Specific	Amount	Kcals	Carb	Prot	Fat	Fibre
red, split, dried, boiled	100g	100	17.5	7.6	0.4	3.3
red, split, dried, boiled	1 tbsp [30g]	30	5.3	2.3	0.1	1.0
Lettuce						
average, raw	100g	14	1.7	0.8	0.5	1.3
average, raw	1 serving [30g]	4	0.5	0.2	0.2	0.4
Iceberg, raw	100g	13	1.9	0.7	0.3	1.3
Iceberg, raw	1 serving [80g]	10	0.6	0.2	0.1	0.4
Marrow						
boiled	100g	9	1.6	0.4	0.2	1.0
raw	100g	12	2.2	0.5	0.2	1.1
Mushrooms						
boiled	100g	11	0.4	1.8	0.3	2.3
raw	100g	15	0.4	1.8	0.5	2.3
raw	1, average [10g]	1	trace	0.2	trace	0.2
Mustard and Cress						
raw	100g	13	0.4	1.6	0.6	3.3
raw	1 punnet [40g]	5	0.2	0.6	0.2	1.3
Okra						
boiled	100g	28	2.7	2.5	0.9	4.1
raw	100g	31	3.0	2.8	1.0	4.5
raw	10, medium [50g]	16	1.5	1.4	0.5	2.3
Onions						
boiled	100g	17	3.7	0.6	0.1	0.7
cocktail/ silverskin, drained	100g	15	3.1	0.6	0.1	0.6

Specific	Amount	Kcals	Carb	Prot	Fat	Fibre
pickled, drained	100g	24	4.9	0.9	0.2	1.3
pickled, drained	1, average [10g]	2	0.5	0.1	trace	0.1
raw	100g	36	7.9	1.2	0.2	1.5
raw	1, average [90g]	32	7.1	1.1	0.2	1.4
raw	1 slice [20g]	7	1.6	0.2	trace	0.3
Parsnip						
boiled	100g	66	12.9	1.6	1.2	4.4
raw	100g	64	12.5	1.8	1.1	4.3
Peas						
boiled	100g	79	10.0	6.7	1.6	4.7
frozen, boiled	100g	69	9.7	6.0	0.9	7.3
Mange-tout, boiled	100g	261	3.3	3.2	0.1	4.0
Mange-tout, raw	100g	32	4.2	3.6	0.2	4.2
Petits pois, frozen, boiled	100g	49	5.5	5.0	0.9	6.4
raw	100g	83	11.3	6.9	1.5	4.7
Peppers						
green, boiled	100g	18	2.6	1.0	0.5	2.1
green, raw	100g	15	2.6	0.8	0.3	1.9
green, raw	1, medium [160g]	24	4.2	1.3	0.5	3.0
green, raw	1 sliced ring [10g]	2	0.3	0.1	trace	0.2
red, boiled	100g	34	7.0	1.1	0.4	2.1
red, raw	100g	32	6.4	1.0	0.4	1.9
red, raw	1, medium [160g]	51	10.2	1.6	0.6	3.0
red, raw	1 sliced ring [10g]	3	0.6	0.1	trace	0.2

Specific	Amount	Kcals	Carb	Prot	Fat	Fibre
mixed, raw	100g	20	0.7	2.9	0.6	1.9
Plantain						
boiled	100g	112	28.5	0.8	0.2	2.2
raw	100g	117	29.4	1.1	0.3	2.3
Potatoes (Chips)						
fine cut, frozen, fried in oil	100g	364	41.2	4.5	21.3	4.0
homemade, fried in oil	100g	189	30.1	3.9	6.7	3.0
oven, frozen, baked	100g	162	29.8	3.2	4.2	2.8
chip shop, fried in oil	1 serving [200g]	478	61.0	6.4	24.8	6.0
straight cut, frozen, fried in oil	100g	273	36.0	4.1	13.5	3.5
Potatoes (New)						
boiled	100g	75	17.8	1.5	0.3	1.2
boiled in skins	100g	66	15.4	1.4	0.3	1.3
raw	100g	70	16.1	1.7	0.3	1.3
Potatoes (Old)						
baked, flesh and skin	100g	136	31.7	3.9	0.2	2.7
baked, flesh and skin	1 medium-size [180g]	245	57.1	7.0	0.4	4.9
boiled	100g	72	17.0	1.8	0.1	1.2
raw	100g	75	17.2	2.1	0.2	1.6
Pumpkin						
raw	100g	13	2.2	0.7	0.2	0.5
boiled	100g	13	2.1	0.6	0.3	0.5

Specific	Amount	Kcals	Carb	Prot	Fat	Fibre
Radish						
raw	100g	12	1.9	0.7	0.2	0.9
raw	1, average [10g]	1	0.2	0.1	trace	0.1
Spinach						
boiled	100g	19	0.8	2.2	0.8	3.1
frozen, boiled	100g	21	0.5	3.1	0.8	3.1
raw	100g	25	1.6	2.8	0.8	3.9
Spring greens						
boiled	100g	20	1.6	1.9	0.7	3.4
raw	100g	33	3.1	3.0	1.0	6.1
Spring onions						
raw	100g	23	3.0	2.0	0.5	1.5
raw	1, average [20g]	5	0.6	0.4	0.1	0.3
Swede						
raw	100g	24	5.0	0.7	0.3	2.4
boiled	100g	11	2.3	0.3	0.1	1.2
Sweet potato						
boiled	100g	84	20.5	1.1	0.3	2.1
raw	100g	87	21.3	1.2	0.3	2.3
Sweetcorn						
baby, canned, drained	100g	23	2.0	2.9	0.4	1.5
kernels, canned, drained	100g	122	26.6	2.9	1.2	3.9
kernels, canned, drained	1 tbsp [30g]	37	8.0	0.9	0.4	1.2
on-the-cob, whole, boiled	100g	66	11.6	2.5	1.4	2.5

Specific	Amount	Kcals	Carb	Prot	Fat	Fibre
on-the-cob, whole, boiled	1, kernels only [125g]	83	14.5	3.1	1.8	3.1
Tomatoes						
canned, with juice	100g	16	3.0	1.0	0.1	0.8
grilled	100g	49	8.9	2.0	0.9	3.7
raw	100g	17	3.1	0.7	0.3	1.3
Turnip						
boiled	100g	12	2.0	0.6	0.2	2.0
raw	100g	23	4.7	0.9	0.3	2.5
Watercress						
raw	100g	22	0.4	3.0	1.0	3.0
raw	1 bunch [80g]	18	0.3	2.4	0.8	2.4
Yam						
boiled	100g	133	33.0	1.7	0.3	3.5
boiled	1, medium [130g]	173	42.9	2.2	0.4	4.6

Nuts and Seeds

Specific	Amount	Kcals	Carb	Prot	Fat	Fibre
Almonds	100g	612	6.9	21.1	55.8	12.9
	6 whole [10g]	61	0.7	2.1	5.6	1.3
Brazil nuts	100g	682	3.1	14.1	68.2	8.1
	6 whole [20g]	136	0.6	2.8	13.6	1.6
Cashew nuts						
roasted, salted	100g	611	18.8	20.5	50.9	3.2
roasted, salted	10 whole [10g]	61	1.9	2.1	5.1	0.3
roasted, salted	25g packet	153	4.7	5.1	12.7	0.8
Chestnuts	100g	170	36.6	2.0	2.7	6.1
	5 whole [50g]	85	18.3	1.0	1.4	3.0
Coconut						
creamed, block	100g	669	7.0	6.0	68.8	N
dessicated	100g	604	6.4	5.6	62.0	21.1
Hazelnuts	100g	650	6.0	14.1	63.5	8.9
	10 whole [10g]	65	0.6	1.4	6.4	0.9
Macadamia nuts						
salted	100g	748	4.8	7.9	77.6	5.3
salted	6 nuts [10g]	75	0.5	0.8	7.8	0.5
Mixed nuts	100g	607	7.9	22.9	54.1	7.5
	40g packet	243	3.2	9.2	21.6	3.0
	50g packet	304	4.0	11.5	27.1	3.8

Specific	Amount	Kcals	Carb	Prot	Fat	Fibre
Peanuts						
plain	100g	564	12.5	25.6	46.1	7.3
plain	10 whole [10g]	56	1.3	2.6	4.6	0.7
roasted, salted	100g	602	7.1	24.5	53.0	6.9
roasted, salted	10 whole [10g]	60	0.7	2.5	5.3	0.7
roasted, salted	25g packet	151	1.8	6.1	13.3	1.7
roasted, salted	40g packet	241	2.8	9.8	21	2.8
roasted, salted	50g packet	301	3.6	12.3	26.5	3.5
dry roasted	100g	589	10.3	25.5	49.8	7.4
Pecan nuts	100g	689	5.8	9.2	70.1	4.7
	3 nuts [18g]	124	1.0	1.7	12.6	0.8
Pine nuts	100g	688	4.0	14.0	68.6	1.9
Pistachio nuts	100g	331	4.6	9.9	30.5	3.3
	10 nuts [8g]	26	0.4	0.8	2.4	0.3
Walnuts	100g	688	3.3	14.7	68.5	5.9
	6 halves [20g]	138	0.7	2.9	13.7	1.2
	for bread [12g]	75	1.6	2.7	6.4	0.8
Sesame seeds	100g	578	0.9	18.2	58.0	7.9
	1 tbsp [10g]	58	0.1	1.8	5.8	0.8
Sunflower seeds	100g	581	18.6	19.8	47.5	6.0
	1 tbsp [14g]	81	2.6	2.8	6.7	0.8

Cereals

Specific	Amount	Kcals	Carb	Prot	Fat	Fibre
Bran						
Wheat	100g	206	26.8	14.1	5.5	39.6
Wheat	1 tbsp [7g]	14	1.9	1.0	0.4	2.7
Bread						
Brown, average	100g	218	44.3	8.5	2.0	5.9
Brown, average	25g slice	55	1.8	2.0	0.5	1.5
Croissants	100g	360	38.3	8.3	20.3	2.5
Granary	100g	235	46.3	9.3	2.7	6.5
Granary	25g slice	59	11.6	2.3	0.7	1.6
Hovis	100g	212	41.5	9.5	2.0	5.1
Hovis	25g slice	53	10.4	2.4	0.5	1.3
Malt	100g	268	56.8	8.3	2.4	6.5
Malt	35g slice	93.8	19.9	2.9	0.8	2.3
Pitta	100g	265	57.9	9.2	1.2	3.9
Pitta	75g pitta	199	43.4	6.9	0.9	2.9
Pitta	95g pitta	252	55.0	8.7	1.1	3.7
Rolls, brown, crusty	100g	255	50.4	10.3	2.8	7.1
Rolls, brown, crusty	1 roll [48g]	122	22.7	4.9	1.3	3.4
Rolls, brown, soft	100g	268	51.8	10.0	2.8	6.4
Rolls, brown, soft	1 roll [43g]	115	22.3	4.3	1.2	2.8
Rolls, hamburger buns	100g	264	48.8	9.1	5.0	4.0

Specific	Amount	Kcals	Carb	Prot	Fat	Fibre
Rolls, hamburger buns	1 roll [50g]	132	24.4	4.6	2.5	2.0
Rolls, white, crusty	100g	280	57.6	10.9	2.3	4.3
Rolls, white, crusty	1 roll [50g]	140	28.8	5.5	1.2	2.2
Rolls, white, soft	100g	268	51.6	9.2	4.2	3.9
Rolls, white, soft	1 roll [45g]	121	23.2	4.4	1.9	1.8
Rolls, wholemeal	100g	241	48.3	9.0	2.9	8.8
Rolls, wholemeal	1 roll [45g]	108	21.7	4.1	1.3	4.0
Rye	100g	219	45.8	8.3	1.7	5.8
Rye	25g slice	55	11.5	2.1	0.4	1.5
White, average	100g	235	49.3	8.4	1.9	1.5
White, average	25g slice	59	12.3	2.1	0.5	0.4
Wholemeal, average	100g	215	41.6	9.2	2.5	5.8
Wholemeal, average	25g slice	54	10.4	2.3	0.6	1.5
Custard powder	100g	354	92.0	0.6	0.7	0.1
Flour						
Chapati brown	100g	333	73.7	11.5	1.2	10.3
Chapati, brown	1 level tbsp [20g]	66.6	14.7	2.3	0.2	2.1
Chapati white	100g	335	77.6	9.8	0.5	4.1
Chapati, white	1 level tbsp [20g]	67	15.5	2.0	0.1	0.8
Cornflour	100g	354	92.0	0.6	0.7	0.1
Cornflour	1 level tbsp [20g]	71	18	0.1	0.1	trace
Rye flour	100g	335	75.9	8.2	2.0	11.7
Rye flour	1 level tbsp [20g]	67	15.2	1.6	0.4	2.3
Soya, full fat	100g	447	23.5	36.8	23.5	10.7

Specific	Amount	Kcals	Carb	Prot	Fat	Fibre
Soya, full fat	1 level tbsp [20g]	89	4.7	7.4	4.7	2.1
Soya, low fat	100g	352	28.2	45.3	7.2	13.3
Soya, low fat	1 level tbsp [20g]	70	5.6	9.1	1.4	2.7
Wheat , brown	100g	323	68.5	12.6	1.8	7.0
Wheat, brown	1 level tbsp [20g]	65	13.7	2.5	0.4	1.4
Wheat, white, breadmaking	100g	341	75.3	11.5	1.4	3.7
Wheat, white, breadmaking	1 level tbsp [20g]	68	15.1	2.3	0.5	0.7
Wheat, white, plain	100g	341	77.7	9.4	1.3	3.6
Wheat, white, plain	1 level tbsp [20g]	68	15.5	1.9	0.3	0.7
Wheat, white, self-raising	100g	330	75.6	8.9	1.2	4.1
Wheat, white, self-raising	1 level tbsp [20g]	66	15.1	1.8	0.2	0.8
Wheat, wholemeal	100g	310	63.9	12.7	2.2	8.6
Wheat, wholemeal	1 level tbsp [20g]	62	12.8	2.5	0.4	1.7
Noodles						
Egg, raw	100g	391	71.7	12.1	8.2	5.0
Egg, boiled	100g	62	13.0	2.2	0.5	1.0
Egg, boiled	300g packet	186	39	6.6	1.5	3.0
Wheat, raw	100g	388				
Wheat, boiled	100g	62				
Oatmeal						
raw	100g	375	66.0	11.2	9.2	6.8
Pasta						
Macaroni, raw	100g	348	75.8	12.0	1.8	5.0
Macaroni, boiled	100g	86	18.5	3.0	0.5	1.5

Specific	Amount	Kcals	Carb	Prot	Fat	Fibre
Spaghetti, white, raw	100g	342	74.1	12.0	1.8	5.1
Spaghetti, white, boiled	100g	104	22.2	3.6	0.7	1.8
Spaghetti, wholemeal, raw	100g	324	66.2	13.4	2.5	11.5
Spaghetti, wholemeal, boiled	100g	113	23.2	4.7	0.9	4.0
Fresh egg pasta	100g	270	49.9	10.5	3.2	1.5
Fresh spinach pasta	100g	278	50.9	10.6	3.5	1.5
Dried spinach pasta	100g	36.7	75.2	12.8	1.7	1.5
Rice						
Brown, raw	100g	357	81.3	6.7	2.8	3.8
Brown, boiled	100g	141	32.1	2.6	1.1	1.5
White, easy cook, raw	100g	383	85.8	7.3	3.6	2.7
White, easy cook, boiled	100g	138	30.9	2.6	1.3	1.0
Sago						
raw	100g	355	94.0	0.2	0.2	0.5
Tapioca						
raw	100g	359	95.0	0.4	0.1	0.4
Wheatgerm	100g	357	44.7	26.7	9.2	15.6

Eggs and Dairy Products

Specific	Amount	Kcals	Carb	Prot	Fat	Fibre
Chicken egg						
boiled	100g	147	trace	12.5	10.8	0
boiled	1, size 1 [67g]	98	trace	8.4	7.2	0
boiled	1, size 2 [61g]	90	trace	7.6	6.6	0
boiled	1, size 3 [57g]	84	trace	7.1	6.2	0
boiled	1, size 4 [47g]	69	trace	5.9	5.1	0
white, raw	100g	36	trace	9.0	trace	0
whole, raw	100g	147	trace	12.5	10.8	0
whole, raw	1, size 1 [67g]	98	trace	8.4	7.2	0
whole, raw	1, size 2 [61g]	90	trace	7.6	6.6	0
whole, raw	1, size 3 [57g]	84	trace	7.1	6.2	0
whole, raw	1, size 4 [47g]	69	trace	5.9	5.1	0
yolk, raw	100g	339	trace	16.1	30.5	0
Duck egg						
whole, raw	100g	163	trace	14.3	11.8	0
whole, raw	1, average [75g]	122	trace	17.2	14.2	0
Butter	100g	737	trace	0.5	81.7	0
	7g portion	52	trace	trace	2.9	0
	12g portion	88	trace	0.1	9.8	0
Cheese						
Brie	100g	319	trace	19.3	26.9	0

Specific	Amount	Kcals	Carb	Prot	Fat	Fibre
Camembert	100g	297	trace	20.9	23.7	0
Cheddar, average	100g	412	0.1	25.5	34.4	0
Cheddar, vegetarian	100g	425	trace	25.8	35.7	0
Cheddar-type, reduced fat	100g	261	trace	31.5	15.0	0
Cheese spread	100g	276	4.4	13.5	22.8	0
Cottage cheese, plain	100g	98	2.1	13.8	3.9	0
Cottage cheese, reduced fat	100g	78	3.3	13.3	1.4	0
Cottage cheese, with additions	100g	95	2.6	12.8	3.8	trace
Cream cheese	100g	439	trace	3.1	47.4	0
Danish Blue	100g	347	trace	20.1	29.6	0
Dolcellate	100g	320	0.2	19.2	27	0
Edam	100g	333	trace	26.0	25.4	trace
Emmental	100g	401	trace	29	31.4	trace
Feta	100g	250	1.5	15.6	20.2	0
Fromage Frais, fruit	100g	131	13.8	6.8	5.8	trace
Fromage Frais, fruit	60g pot	79	8.3	4.1	3.5	trace
Fromage Frais, plain	100g	113	5.7	6.8	7.1	0
Fromage Frais, plain	60g pot	68	3.4	4.1	4.3	0
Fromage Frais, very low fat	100g	58	6.8	7.7	0.2	trace
Fromage Frais, very low fat	60g pot	35	4.1	4.6	0.1	trace
Gouda	100g	375	trace	24.0	31.0	0
Hard cheese, average	100g	405	0.1	24.7	34.0	0
Parmesan	100g	452	trace	39.4	32.7	0
Processed, plain	100g	330	0.9	20.8	27.0	0

Specific	Amount	Kcals	Carb	Prot	Fat	Fibre
Soft cheese, full fat	100g	313	trace	8.6	31.0	0
Soft cheese, medium fat	100g	179	3.1	9.2	14.5	0
Stilton	100g	411	0.1	22.7	35.5	0
White, average	100g	376	0.1	23.4	31.3	0
Cream, fresh						
clotted	100g	586	2.3	1.6	63.5	0
clotted	small carton [150g]	879	3.5	2.4	95.3	0
double	100g	449	2.7	1.7	48.0	0
double	small carton [150g]	674	4.1	2.6	72.0	0
half	100g	148	4.3	3.0	13.3	0
half	small carton [150g]	222	6.5	4.5	20.0	0
single	100g	198	4.1	2.6	19.1	0
single	small carton [150g]	297	6.2	3.9	28.7	0
soured	100g	205	3.8	2.9	19.9	0
soured	small carton [150g]	308	5.7	4.4	30.0	0
whipping	100g	373	3.1	2.0	39.3	0
whipping	small carton [150g]	560	4.7	3.0	59.0	0
Cream, sterilized						
canned	100g	239	3.7	2.5	23.9	0
Dairy/Fat spread	100g	662	trace	0.4	73.4	0
	10g portion	66	trace	trace	7.3	0
Milk, evaporated						
whole	100g	151	8.5	8.4	9.4	0
whole	170g can	257	14.5	14.3	16.0	0

Specific	Amount	Kcals	Carb	Prot	Fat	Fibre
Milk, goat's						
pasteurized	100g	60	4.4	3.1	3.5	0
pasteurized	1 pint [585g]	351	25.7	18.1	20.5	0
Milk, semi-skimmed						
pasteurized	100g	46	5.0	3.3	1.6	0
pasteurized	1 pint [585g]	269	29.3	19.3	9.4	0
pasteurized	30g portion for tea/coffee	14	1.5	1.0	0.5	0
fortified plus smp	100g	51	5.8	3.7	1.6	0
fortified plus smp	1 pint [585g]	298	33.9	21.6	9.4	0
UHT	100g	46	4.8	3.3	1.7	0
UHT	1 pint [585g]	269	28.1	19.3	9.9	0
Milk, sheep's						
raw	100g	95	5.1	5.4	6.0	0
raw	1 pint [585g]	556	29.8	31.6	35.1	0
pasteurized	100g	33	5.0	3.3	0.1	0
pasteurized	1 pint [585g]	193	29.3	19.3	0	0
Milk, skimmed						
pasteurized	30g portion for tea or coffee	10	1.5	1.0	trace	0
fortified plus smp	100g	39	6.0	3.8	0.1	0
fortified plus smp	1 pint [585g]	228	35.1	22.2	0.6	0
UHT, fortified	100g	35	5.0	3.5	0.2	0

Specific	Amount	Kcals	Carb	Prot	Fat	Fibre
Milk, soya						
plain, unsweetened	100g	32	0.8	2.9	1.9	0
plain, unsweetened	1 pint [585g]	187	4.7	17.0	11.1	0
Milk, whole						
pasteurized	100g	66	4.8	3.2	3.9	0
pasteurized	1 pint [585g]	386	28.1	18.7	22.8	0
pasteurized	30g portion for tea or coffee	20	1.4	1.0	1.2	0
sterilized	100g	66	4.5	3.5	3.9	0
sterilized	1 pint [585g]	386	26.3	20.5	22.8	0
UHT, fortified	1 pint [585g]	205	29.3	20.5	1.2	0
Yoghurt						
Greek, cows	100g	115	2.0	6.4	9.1	0
Greek, sheep's	100g	106	5.6	4.4	7.5	0
Low fat, flavoured	100g	90	17.9	3.8	0.9	0
Low fat, fruit	100g	90	17.9	4.1	0.7	trace
Low fat, plain	100g	56	7.5	5.1	0.8	0
Soya	100g	72	3.9	5.0	4.2	0
Whole milk, fruit	100g	105	15.7	5.1	2.8	trace
Whole milk, plain	100g	79	7.8	5.7	3.0	0
Whole milk, plain	150g carton	119	11.7	8.6	4.5	0

Meat

Specific	Amount	Kcals	Carb	Prot	Fat	Fibre
Bacon						
Collar joint, boiled	100g	325	0	20.4	27.0	0
Collar joint, raw	100g	319	0	14.6	28.9	0
Gammon joint, boiled	100g	269	0	24.7	18.9	0
Gammon joint, raw	100g	236	0	17.6	18.3	0
Gammon rasher, grilled	100g	228	0	29.5	12.2	0
Rasher [back], grilled	1 rasher [25g]	101	0	6.3	8.5	0
Rasher [back], raw	100g	428	0	14.2	41.2	0
Rasher [middle], grilled	1 rasher [40g]	166	0	10.0	14.0	0
Rasher [middle], raw	100g	425	0	14.3	40.9	0
Rasher [streaky], grilled	1 rasher [20g]	84	0	4.9	7.2	0
Rasher [streaky], raw	100g	414	0	14.6	39.5	0
Beef						
Brisket, boiled	100g	326	0	27.6	23.9	0
Brisket, raw	100g	252	0	16.8	20.5	0
Forerib, raw	100g	290	0	16.0	25.1	0
Forerib, roast	100g	349	0	22.4	28.8	0
Mince, raw	100g	221	0	18.8	16.2	0
Mince, stewed	100g	229	0	23.1	15.2	0
Rump steak, grilled	100g	218	0	27.3	12.1	0
Rump steak, raw	100g	197	0	18.9	13.5	0

Specific	Amount	Kcals	Carb	Prot	Fat	Fibre
Salted	100g	119	0	27.1	0.4	0
Silverside, salted, boiled	100g	242	0	28.6	14.2	0
Sirloin, raw	100g	272	0	16.6	22.8	0
Sirloin, roast	100g	284	0	23.6	21.1	0
Stewing steak, raw	100g	176	0	20.2	10.6	0
Stewing steak, stewed	100g	223	0	30.9	11.0	0
Topside, raw	100g	179	0	19.6	11.2	0
Topside, roast	100g	214	0	26.6	12.0	0
Chicken						
Dark meat, boiled	100g	204	0	28.6	9.9	0
Dark meat, raw	100g	126	0	19.1	5.5	0
Dark meat, roast	100g	155	0	23.1	6.9	0
Leg quarter, roast	100g	92	0	15.4	3.4	0
Light and dark meat, boiled	100g	183	0	29.2	7.3	0
Light and dark meat, raw	100g	121	0	20.5	4.3	0
Light and dark meat, roast	100g	148	0	24.8	5.4	0
Light meat, boiled	100g	163	0	29.7	4.9	0
Light meat, raw	100g	116	0	21.8	3.2	0
Light meat, roast	100g	142	0	26.5	4.0	0
Wing quarter, roast	100g	74	0	12.4	2.7	0
Duck						
raw	100g	122	0	19.7	4.8	0
roast	100g	189	0	25.3	9.7	0

Specific	Amount	Kcals	Carb	Prot	Fat	Fibre
Goose						
roast	100g	319	0	29.3	22.4	0
Grouse						
roast	100g	173	0	31.3	5.3	0
roast	1 grouse [160g]	277	0	50.1	8.5	0
Ham						
Honey roast	100g	108	2.4	18.2	2.9	0
Honey roast	30g slice	32	0.7	5.4	0.9	0
Smoked	100g	94	0.8	17.6	2.3	0
Smoked	30g slice	28	0.2	5.9	0.7	0
Hare						
Stewed	100g	192	0	29.9	8.0	0
Lamb						
Breast, raw	100g	378	0	16.7	34.6	0
Breast, roast	100g	410	0	19.1	37.1	0
Chops, Loin, grilled	100g	355	0	23.5	29.0	0
Chops, Loin, grilled	1 chop [90g]	320	0	21.2	26.1	0
Chops, Loin, raw	100g	377	0	14.6	35.4	0
Cutlets, grilled	100g	370	0	23.0	30.9	0
Cutlets, grilled	1 cutlet [50g]	185	0	11.5	15.5	0
Cutlets, raw	100g	386	0	14.7	36.3	0
Leg, raw	100g	240	0	17.9	18.7	0
Leg, roast	100g	266	0	26.1	17.9	0
Scrag and neck, raw	100g	316	0	15.6	28.2	0

Specific	Amount	Kcals	Carb	Prot	Fat	Fibre
Scrag and neck, stewed	100g	292	0	25.6	21.1	0
Shoulder, raw	100g	314	0	15.6	28.0	0
Shoulder, roast	100g	316	0	19.9	26.3	0
Heart, lamb, raw	100g	119	0	17.1	5.6	0
Heart, ox, raw	100g	108	0	18.9	3.6	0
Heart, ox, stewed	100g	179	0	31.4	5.9	0
Heart, sheep, roast	100g	237	0	26.1	14.7	0
Kidney, lamb, raw	100g	90	0	16.5	2.7	0
Kidney, ox, raw	100g	86	0	15.7	2.6	0
Kidney, pig, raw	100g	90	0	16.3	2.7	0
Liver, calf, raw	100g	153	1.9	20.1	7.3	0
Liver, chicken, raw	100g	135	0.6	19.1	6.3	0
Liver, lamb, raw	100g	179	1.6	20.1	10.3	0
Liver, ox raw	100g	163	2.2	21.1	7.8	0
Liver, pig, raw	100g	154	2.1	21.3	6.8	0
Oxtail, stewed	100g	243	0	30.5	13.4	0
Sweetbread, lamb, raw	100g	131	0	15.3	7.8	0
Tongue, lamb, raw	100g	193	0	15.3	14.6	0
Tongue, ox, boiled	100g	293	0	19.5	23.9	0
Tongue, ox, pickled, raw	100g	220	0	15.7	17.5	0
Tongue, sheep, stewed	100g	289	0	18.2	24.0	0
Tripe, dressed	100g	60	0	9.4	2.5	0
Partridge						
roast	100g	212	0	36.7	7.2	0

Specific	Amount	Kcals	Carb	Prot	Fat	Fibre
roast	1 partridge [260g]	551	0	95.4	18.7	0
Pheasant						
roast	100g	213	0	32.2	9.3	0
roast	1 pheasant [430g]	916	0	138.5	40.0	0
Pigeon						
roast	100g	230	0	27.8	13.2	0
roast	1 pigeon [115g]	265	0	32.0	15.2	0
Pork						
Belly rashers, grilled	100g	398	0	21.1	34.8	0
Belly rashers, raw	100g	381	0	15.3	35.5	0
Chops, Loin, grilled	100g	332	0	28.5	24.2	0
Chops, Loin, raw	100g	329	0	15.9	29.5	0
Leg, raw	100g	269	0	16.6	22.5	0
Leg, roast	100g	286	0	26.9	19.8	0
Trotters and tails, boiled	100g	280	0	19.8	22.3	0
Rabbit						
raw	100g	124	0	21.9	4.0	0
stewed	100g	179	0	27.3	7.7	0
Tongue						
canned	100g	213	0	16.0	16.5	0
Turkey						
Dark meat, raw	100g	114	0	20.3	3.6	0
Dark meat, roast	100g	148	0	27.8	4.1	0
Light and dark meat, raw	100g	107	0	21.9	2.2	0

Specific	Amount	Kcals	Carb	Prot	Fat	Fibre
Light and dark meat, roast	100g	140	0	28.8	2.7	0
Light meat, raw	100g	103	0	23.2	1.1	0
Light meat, roast	100g	132	0	29.8	1.4	0
Veal						
Fillet, raw	100g	109	0	21.1	2.7	0
Fillet, roast	100g	230	0	31.6	11.5	0
Venison						
Haunch, roast	100g	198	0	35.0	6.4	0
Haunch, roast	120g portion	238	0	42.0	7.7	0

Fish and Seafood

Specific	Amount	Kcals	Carb	Prot	Fat	Fibre
Anchovies						
canned in oil, drained	100g	280	0	25.2	19.9	0
canned in oil, drained	1 anchovy [3g]	8.4	0	0.8	0.6	0
Cockles						
boiled	100g	48	trace	11.3	0.3	0
boiled	1 cockle [4g]	2	0	0.5	trace	0
Cod						
dried, salted, boiled	100g	138	0	32.5	0.9	0
Fillets, baked	100g	96	0	21.4	1.2	0
Fillets, raw	100g	76	0	17.4	0.7	0
Steaks, frozen, raw,	100g	68	0	15.6	0.6	0
Crab						
boiled	100g	127	0	20.1	5.2	0
Haddock						
fillet, raw	100g	73	0	16.8	0.6	0
middle cut, steamed	100g	98	0	22.8	0.8	0
middle cut, steamed	85g portion	83	0	19.4	0.7	0
smoked, steamed	100g	101	0	23.3	0.9	0
smoked, steamed	85g portion	86	5.2	19.8	0.8	0
middle cut, steamed	100g	98	0	22.8	0.8	0

Specific	Amount	Kcals	Carb	Prot	Fat	Fibre
Halibut						
middle cut, steamed	100g	83	0	19.4	0.7	0
raw	100g	92	0	17.7	2.4	0
Herring						
grilled	100g	135	0	13.9	8.8	0
raw	100g	234	0	16.8	18.5	0
Kipper						
baked	100g	205	0	25.5	11.4	0
Lemon sole						
raw	100g	81	0	17.1	1.4	0
steamed	100g	91	0	20.6	0.9	0
Lobster						
boiled	100g	119	0	22.1	3.4	0
Mackerel						
fried	100g	188	0	21.5	11.3	0
raw	100g	223	0	19.0	16.3	0
smoked	100g	354	0	18.9	30.9	0
Mussels						
boiled	100g	87	trace	17.2	2.0	0
boiled	1 mussel [7g]	6.1	trace	1.2	0.1	0
Pilchards						
in tomato sauce, canned	100g	126	0.7	18.8	5.4	trace
in tomato sauce, canned	1 pilchard [55g]	69.3	0.4	10.3	3.0	trace

Specific	Amount	Kcals	Carb	Prot	Fat	Fibre
Plaice						
raw	100g	91	0	17.9	2.2	0
steamed	100g	93	0	18.9	1.9	0
Prawns						
boiled	100g	107	0	22.6	1.8	0
boiled	1 prawn [3g]	3	0	0.7	0.1	0
Saithe						
raw	100g	73	0	17.0	0.5	0
steamed	100g	99	0	23.3	0.6	0
Salmon						
raw	100g	182	0	18.4	12.0	0
smoked	100g	142	0	25.4	4.5	0
steamed	100g	197	0	20.1	13.0	0
Sardines						
in oil, canned, drained	100g	217	0	23.7	13.6	0
in oil, canned, drained	1 sardine [25g]	54.3	0	5.9	3.4	0
in tomato sauce, canned	100g	177	0.5	17.8	11.6	trace
Scampi						
in breadcrumbs, fried	100g	316	28.9	12.2	17.6	1.1
in breadcrumbs, fried	1 piece [15g]	79	7.2	3.1	4.4	0.2
Shrimps						
frozen	100g	73	0	16.5	0.8	0
Skate						
in batter, fried	100g	199	4.9	17.9	12.1	0.2

Specific	Amount	Kcals	Carb	Prot	Fat	Fibre
Squid						
frozen, raw	100g	66	0	13.1	1.5	0
Trout						
Brown, steamed	100g	135	0	23.5	4.5	0
Tuna						
in brine, canned, drained	100g	99	0	23.5	0.6	0
in oil, canned, drained	100g	189	0	27.1	9.0	0
Whelks						
boiled, weighed with shell	100g	14	trace	2.8	0.3	0
Whitebait						
rolled in flour, fried	100g	525	5.3	19.5	47.5	0.2
rolled in flour, fried	1 whole	21	0.2	0.8	1.9	trace
Whiting						
steamed	100g	92	0	20.9	0.9	0
steamed	85g portion	78	0	17.8	0.8	0
Winkles						
boiled, weighed with shell	100g	14	trace	2.9	0.3	0

Fats and Oils

Specific	Amount	Kcals	Carb	Prot	Fat	Fibre
Animal fat						
Dripping, beef	100g	891	trace	trace	99.0	0
Lard	100g	891	trace	trace	99.0	0
Suet, shredded	100g	826	12.1	trace	86.7	0.6
Ghee						
Vegetable	100g	898	trace	trace	99.8	0
Oil						
Coconut oil	100g	899	0	trace	99.9	0
Olive oil	100g	899	0	trace	99.9	0
Palm oil	100g	899	0	trace	99.9	0
Peanut oil	100g	899	0	trace	99.9	0
Safflower oil	100g	899	0	trace	99.9	0
Sesame oil	100g	881	0	0.2	99.7	0
Soya oil	100g	899	0	trace	99.9	0
Sunflower seed oil	100g	899	0	trace	99.9	0
Vegetable oil, blended, average	100g	899	0	trace	99.9	0
Spreading fat						
Butter	100g	737	trace	0.5	81.7	0
Dairy/fat spread	100g	662	trace	0.4	73.4	0
Low fat spread	100g	390	0.5	5.8	40.5	0
Margarine, polyunsaturated	100g	739	1.0	0.2	81.6	0

Confectionery and Snacks

Specific	Amount	Kcals	Carb	Prot	Fat	Fibre
Chocolate						
Chocolate, milk	100g	529	59.4	8.4	30.3	N
Chocolate, plain	100g	525	64.8	4.7	29.2	N
Chocolate, white	100g	529	58.3	8.0	30.9	N
Chocolates, fancy and filled [assorted]	100g	460	73.3	4.1	18.8	trace
Non-chocolate Confectionery						
Boiled sweets	100g	327	87.3	trace	trace	0
Toffees, mixed	100g	430	71.1	2.1	17.2	0
Savoury Snacks						
Bombay mix	100g	503	35.1	18.8	32.9	6.2
Corn snacks	100g	519	54.3	7.0	31.9	1.0
Peanuts and raisins	100g	435	37.5	15.3	26.0	6.8
Potato crisps, assorted	100g	546	49.3	5.6	37.6	4.3
Potato crisps, assorted	28g bag	153	13.8	1.6	10.5	1.2
Potato crisps, low fat, assorted	100g	456	63.0	6.6	21.5	6.3
Potato crisps, low fat, assorted	28g bag	128	17.6	1.8	6.0	1.8
Potato crisps, thick cut, old style	100g	485	42.7	6.9	31.0	13.9
Potato Hoops	100g	523	58.5	3.9	32.0	N

Sauces and Miscellaneous

Specific	Amount	Kcals	Carb	Prot	Fat	Fibre
Miscellaneous						
Baking powder	100g	163	37.8	5.2	trace	0
Baking powder	1 level tsp	7	1.5	0.2	trace	0
Gelatine	100g	338	0	84	0	0
Salt	100g	0	0	0	0	0
Salt	1 tsp	0	0	0	0	0
Vinegar	100g	4	0.6	0.4	0	0
Vinegar	1 tbsp [15g]	1	0.1	0.1	0	0
Yeast, baker's compressed	100g	5	1.1	11.4	0.4	6.2
Yeast, dried	100g	169	3.5	35.6	1.5	19.7
Salad dressing						
French dressing	100g	649	0.1	0.3	72.1	0
Mayonnaise	100g	691	1.7	1.1	75.6	0
Salad cream	100g	348	16.7	1.5	31.0	N
Salad cream, reduced calorie	100g	194	9.4	1.0	17.2	N
Sauce						
Horseradish sauce	100g	153	17.9	2.5	8.4	2.5
Mint sauce	100g	87	21.5	1.6	trace	N
Soy sauce	100g	64	8.3	8.7	0	0
Soy sauce	1 tsp [5g]	3	0.4	0.4	0	0

Beverages

Specific	Amount	Kcals	Carb	Prot	Fat	Fibre
Ale						
Bottled, brown	100ml	28	3	trace	0	0
Bottled, brown	1 pint	159	17	trace	0	0
Bottled, pale	100ml	32	2	trace	0	0
Bottled, pale	1 pint	182	11.4	trace	0	0
Beer						
Bitter, canned	100ml	32	2.3	trace	0	0
Bitter, canned	1 pint	182	13.1	trace	0	0
Bitter, draught	100ml	32	2.3	trace	0	0
Bitter, draught	1 pint	182	13.1	trace	0	0
Bitter, keg	100ml	31	2.3	trace	0	0
Bitter, keg	1 pint	176	13.1	trace	0	0
Mild, draught	100ml	25	1.6	trace	0	0
Mild, draught	1 pint	142	9.1	trace	0	0
Stout	100ml	37	4.2	trace	0	0
Stout	1 pint	210	23.5	trace	0	0
Stout, extra	100ml	39	2.1	trace	0	0
Stout, extra	1 pint	222	11.9	trace	0	0
Cider						
Dry	100ml	36	2.6	trace	0	0
Dry	1 pint	204	14.8	trace	0	0

Specific	Amount	Kcals	Carb	Prot	Fat	Fibre
Sweet	100ml	42	4.3	trace	0	0
Sweet	1 pint	238	24.4	trace	0	0
Vintage	100ml	101	7.3	trace	0	0
Vintage	1 pint	573	41.5	trace	0	0
Fortified Wine						
Port	30ml	47	3.6	trace	0	0
Sherry, dry	30ml	35	0.5	trace	0	0
Sherry, medium	30ml	35	1.0	trace	0	0
Sherry, sweet	30ml	43	2	trace	0	0
Lager						
Bottled	100ml	29	1.5	trace	0	0
Bottled	1 pint	165	8.5	trace	0	0
Spirits						
Brandy, 40% proof	30ml	65	trace	trace	0	0
Gin, 40% proof	30ml	65	trace	trace	0	0
Rum, 40% proof	30ml	65	trace	trace	0	0
Vodka, 40% proof	30ml	65	trace	trace	0	0
Whisky, 40% proof	30ml	65	trace	trace	0	0
Wine						
Red	100ml	68	0.3	trace	0	0
Red	1 bottle [750ml]	510	2.3	trace	0	0
Red	1 glass [120ml]	82	0.4	trace	0	0
Rosé, medium	100ml	71	2.5	trace	0	0
Rosé, medium	1 bottle [750ml]	533	18.8	trace	0	0

Specific	Amount	Kcals	Carb	Prot	Fat	Fibre
Rosé, medium	1 glass [120ml]	85	3.0	trace	0	0
White, dry	100ml	66	0.6	trace	0	0
White, dry	1 bottle [750ml]	495	4.5	trace	0	0
White, dry	1 glass [120ml]	79	0.7	trace	0	0
White, medium	100ml	75	3.4	trace	0	0
White, medium	1 bottle [750ml]	563	25.5	trace	0	0
White, medium	1 glass [120ml]	90	4.1	trace	0	0
White, sparkling	100ml	76	1.4	trace	0	0
White, sparkling	1 bottle [750ml]	570	10.5	trace	0	0
White, sparkling	1 glass [120ml]	91	1.7	trace	0	0
White, sweet	100ml	94	5.9	trace	0	0
White, sweet	1 bottle [750ml]	705	44.3	trace	0	0
White, sweet	1 glass [120ml]	113	53.2	trace	0	0
Carbonated drink						
Coca-cola	100g	36	10.5	trace	0	0
Coca-cola	can [330g]	119	5.0	trace	0	0
Lemonade, bottled	100g	21	5.6	trace	0	0
Lemonade, bottled	1 glass [200g]	42	11.2	trace	0	0
Cocoa						
powder	100g	312	11.5	18.5	21.7	0.2
powder	4g portion	12.5	0.5	0.7	0.9	trace
Coffee						
Instant, 30g of whole milk	1 mug	22	1.6	1.3	1.2	0
Instant, without milk or sugar	1 mug [260g]	2	0.2	0.3	0	0

Specific	Amount	Kcals	Carb	Prot	Fat	Fibre
Drinking chocolate						
powder	100g	366	77.4	5.5	6.0	N
powder	18g portion	66	14	1.0	1.1	N
Horlicks						
Instant, powder	100g	378	78	12.4	4.0	trace
Instant, powder	25g portion	95	19.5	3.1	1.0	trace
Juice						
Apple juice, unsweetened	100g	38	9.9	0.1	0.1	trace
Apple juice, unsweetened	1 glass [200g]	76	328	0.2	0.2	trace
Grape juice, unsweetened	100g	46	11.7	0.3	0.1	trace
Grape juice, unsweetened	1 glass [200g]	92	23.4	0.6	0.2	trace
Grapefruit juice, unsweetened	100g	33	8.3	0.4	0.1	trace
Grapefruit juice, unsweetened	1 glass [200g]	66	16.6	0.8	0.2	trace
Lemon juice, unsweetened	100g	7	1.6	0.3	trace	0.1
Lemon juice, unsweetened	1 tbsp [15g]	1	0.2	trace	trace	trace
Orange juice, unsweetened	100g	36	8.8	0.5	0.1	0.1
Orange juice, unsweetened	1 glass [200g]	72	17.6	1.0	0.2	0.2
Pineapple juice, unsweetened	100g	41	10.5	0.3	0.1	trace
Pineapple juice, unsweetened	1 glass [200g]	82	21.0	0.6	0.2	trace
Tomato juice	100g	14	3.0	0.8	trace	0.6
Tomato juice	1 glass [200g]	28	6.0	1.6	trace	0.2
Mixers						
Ginger ale	100g	23	5.7	trace	trace	0
Ginger ale	1 glass [200g]	46	11.4	trace	trace	0

Specific	Amount	Kcals	Carb	Prot	Fat	Fibre
Ginger ale, low-calorie	100g	1.8	0.04	trace	trace	0
Ginger ale, low-calorie	220g	3.6	0.08	trace	trace	0
Tonic water	100g	23	5.4	trace	trace	0
Tonic water	1 glass [200g]	46	10.8	trace	trace	0
Tonic water, low-calorie	100g	0.8	trace	trace	trace	0
Tonic water, low-calorie	1 glass [200g]	1.6	trace	trace	trace	0
Ovaltine						
powder	100g	358	79.4	9.0	2.7	trace
powder	25g portion	89	19.8	2.5	1.1	trace
Squash						
Orange drink, undiluted	100g	107	28.5	trace	0	0
Orange drink, undiluted	1 glass [40g]	43	11.4	trace	0	0
Ribena	100g	228	60.8	0.1	0	0
Ribena	1 glass [40g]	91	24.3	trace	0	0
Tea						
No milk or sugar	100g	trace	trace	0.1	trace	0
No milk or sugar	1 cup [200g]	trace	trace	0.2	trace	0
With 30g of whole milk	1 cup [200g]	20	1.4	1.2	1.2	0